The Wellness Kitchen: Savoring Good Health

Cooking Your Way to Optimal Well-Being with Nutrient-Rich Dishes"

By

Mary Ann

2

TABLE OF CONTENTS

Chapter 1

Chapter 2

Chapter 3

Chapter 4

Chapter 5

CHAPTER 1
INTRODUCTION: EMBRACING A WELLNESS-CENTRIC KITCHEN

Greetings from The Wellness Kitchen: Savouring Excellent Health. We delve into the essence of health-focused cuisine on this journey of transformation, where feeding the body becomes an artistic endeavor. Explore the fundamentals of mindful eating, nutritious ingredients, and the thrill of making dishes that not only tantalize your taste buds but also improve your health as we explore the symbiotic relationship between culinary choices and general well-being. Come along on this gastronomic journey towards a bright and well-balanced life.

THE LINK BETWEEN NUTRITION AND WELL-BEING

Nutrition plays a critical role in overall health, affecting physical health, mental clarity, and emotional stability. A balanced diet provides essential nutrients such as vitamins, minerals, proteins, and carbohydrates that are vital for proper functioning of the body.

Proper nutrition promotes physical health by supporting growth, supporting organ health, and strengthening the immune system. Nutrient-dense foods help prevent varieties of health problems, including cardiovascular disease, diabetes, and obesity. Adequate hydration is also important because water is essential for digestion, nutrient absorption, and temperature regulation.

Besides physical health, nutrition has a huge impact on mental health. Certain nutrients play a key role in brain function and neurotransmitter production, affecting mood and cognitive function. For example, omega-3 fatty acids found in fish and nuts are linked to improved cognitive function and reduced risk of depression.

Furthermore, the connection between nutrition and emotional health is clear. Unhealthy eating habits, such as excessive consumption of processed foods or sugary snacks, can lead to energy fluctuations and mood swings. A balanced diet that includes fruits, vegetables, whole grains, and lean proteins promotes a more stable mood and stable energy levels.

Cultural and individual dietary preferences shape dietary choices, underscoring the need for an individualized approach to well-being. Consulting with health professionals or dietitians can help people tailor their diet to suit their specific needs and goals. Ultimately, understanding and prioritizing the relationship between nutrition and well-being is an essential step toward living a healthier, more fulfilling life.

SETTING THE STAGE FOR A HEALTHIER LIFESTYLE

Welcome to The Wellness Kitchen: Enjoying Wellness, where we take you on a journey to pave the way to a healthier lifestyle through thoughtful choices and delicious, nutritious food.

1. A complete culinary adventure

Start by setting health goals. Are you looking for weight control, increased energy, or overall well-being? Plan your culinary adventures around these goals, making sure each meal contributes to your health.

2. Healthy ingredients in the base

The foundation of a healthy lifestyle is the ingredients you choose. Choose fresh, whole foods that are rich in nutrients. Eat a rainbow of fruits, vegetables, lean proteins, and whole grains. Let your kitchen serve as a canvas for colorful and nutritious dishes.

3. Balanced and tasty dishes

Transform your meals into a symphony of flavors by including a balance of essential nutrients. Experiment with herbs and spices to add depth and richness to a dish without relying on too much salt or sugar. Discover the joy of cooking meals that not only nourish your body but also delight your taste buds.

4. Thoughtful Cooking

Mindfulness in the kitchen. Engage your senses while cooking and enjoy every moment. Increase your awareness of portion sizes and listen to your body's hunger and fullness signals. Cooking becomes more than just a task, but a healing ritual that promotes overall health.

5. Attractive atmosphere and positive energy

Pave the way to a healthier lifestyle by creating a welcoming kitchen environment. Surround yourself with positive energy, whether it's upbeat music, natural light, or inspirational quotes. A kitchen that exudes positivity can influence your thinking and strengthen your commitment to a healthy lifestyle.

6. Contacts with family and community

Make the journey to good health a shared experience. Involve family members or friends in cooking as a bonding activity. Exchange recipes, share nutrition ideas, and celebrate the joys of good health together.

7. Educational resources

Gain knowledge about nutrition and health. Research trusted sources, attend seminars, or follow recommendations from trusted health experts. The more informed you are, the better able you will be to make informed choices in your culinary endeavors.

At The Wellness Kitchen, every meal is an opportunity to nourish your body and soul. Through intentional choices, thoughtful practices, and creativity, you're not only paving the way to a healthier lifestyle; You are enjoying the journey to long-term well-being.

CHAPTER 2
STOCKING YOUR WELLNESS KITCHEN

The curvature of wellness food is necessary to develop a nourishing method that supports a healthy lifestyle. Start with full fresh products, such as bright fruits, leafy vegetables, and colored vegetables. Choose organic options when it is possible to reduce the effects of pesticides.

Run proteins such as birds, fish, tofu, and legumes to provide the nutrients needed for muscle health. Select whole grains, such as quinoa, brown rice, and oatmeal for stable energy and fiber. Run many nuts and seeds for more protein, healthy fats, and trace elements.

Emphasizing healthy fats from sources such as avocado, olive oil, and nuts to keep the heart healthy. Keep your kitchen with herbs and spices to add an odor without relying on salt or excessive sugar. Consider the inclusion of turmeric, ginger, and garlic for its potential anti-inflammatory advantages.

Keep a well-equipped store with basic products such as beans, lentils, and whole grain paste for comfortable and nutritious foods. Keep moisturizing, and have a lot of water, herbal tea, and water-filling options.

Invest in high-quality dishes and dishes to make cooking fun. Think about devices such as a juice mixer, and a kitchen that combines grinding and steam for food rich in nutrients. Keep organizing your kitchen to encourage the choice of conscious and deliberate food.

Thinking through the studied healthy kitchen, you create an environment that enhances good health, facilitates the enjoyment of nutrients, and supports the general well.

ESSENTIAL INGREDIENTS FOR NUTRIENT-RICH COOKING

In the wellness kitchen, prioritizing cooking nutrient-rich foods is key to staying healthy. Here are the main ingredients that will enhance the nutritional value of your dishes:

1. **Whole Grains**

Choose whole grains such as quinoa, brown rice, and oats. They contain fiber, vitamins, and minerals to promote digestive health and sustained energy.

2. **Leafy Vegetables**

Add spinach, kale, and chard for more vitamins and minerals. These vegetables are rich in antioxidants that support overall health.

3. **Colorful vegetables**

Includes a variety of colorful vegetables such as bell peppers, carrots, and tomatoes. The different shapes indicate a variety of nutrients, which promotes nutritious nutrition.

4. **Lean Proteins**

Choose lean protein sources such as poultry, fish, tofu, and legumes. Protein is essential for healthy muscles, and these options provide nutrients without excess saturated fat.

5. Healthy Fats

Include healthy sources of fats in your diet, such as avocados, nuts, and olive oil. These fats support heart health and help absorb fat-soluble vitamins.

6. Herbs and Spices

Enhance flavor without adding calories with herbs and spices. Turmeric, garlic, and coriander not only make dishes delicious but also provide potential health benefits.

7. Low Sodium Broth

Choose low sodium broth to help control your salt intake. They are versatile for soups, stews, and cooking grains, adding flavor without excessive sodium.

8. Probiotic foods

These include yogurt, kefir, and fermented vegetables to promote gut health. Probiotics promote the balance of the gut microbiome, which is associated with overall health.

9. Natural Sweeteners

Replace refined sugar with natural sweeteners such as honey or maple syrup in moderation. These options add sweetness and extra nutrients.

10. Nutrient-Rich Snacks

Keep nutrient-rich snacks like raw nuts, seeds, and fruits on hand for convenient, healthy options between meals.

Remember that a balanced combination of these ingredients can transform your kitchen into a hub of delicious and nutritious meals that promote overall health.

ORGANIZING YOUR PANTRY AND FRIDGE FOR SUCCESS

Maintaining a well-organized pantry and refrigerator is a critical step toward success at The Wellness Kitchen. Good health begins with a strategic approach to storing and accessing nutritious ingredients. Here are some tips to help you create an organized culinary haven that promotes well-being.

1. **Classify carefully**

- Separate your pantry and refrigerator into categories such as grains, legumes, canned goods, fresh produce, dairy, and proteins.

- Clearly label shelves or bins so items can be easily found and ensure everything is in its place.

2. **First in, first out (FIFO)**

- Practice the FIFO method to reduce food waste. Arrange items so that old items are in the front and new items are in the back.

- Check expiration dates regularly and throw away expired foods to maintain their freshness and nutritional value.

3. **The main thing is to show up**

- Use clear containers or jars to store grains, nuts, and dried fruits. This improves your vision and reminds you to include these healthy ingredients in your meals.

- Keep frequently used items at eye level for quick access and easier cooking.

4. Careful Meal Planning

- Plan your meals and organize your pantry accordingly. This not only saves time but also encourages healthy food choices.

-Dedicate a designated area for staples such as whole grains, lean proteins, and a variety of colorful vegetables.

5. Smart Storage Solutions

- Invest in storage containers that maximize space and maintain freshness. Consider stackable cereal containers, modular shelves, and adjustable dividers for your refrigerator.

- Use baskets or boxes to group similar items so you can easily get what you need without cluttering the entire space.

6. Thermal zones

- Understand the temperature zones in your refrigerator. Store perishable foods such as dairy and meat in cool places, while fruits and vegetables are best stored in a refrigerator drawer.

- Keep a thermometer in the refrigerator to maintain the ideal temperature for food safety purposes.

7. Regular updates

- Conduct regular pantry and refrigerator checks to assess the condition of ingredients. Get rid of any expired or old items and make a note of what needs replenishing.

- Wipe down shelves and drawers periodically to maintain a clean and healthy environment.

By implementing these organizational strategies, you can transform your pantry and refrigerator into a space that lives up to The Wellness Kitchen's principles. Enjoying good health becomes easier when you can easily access nutritious ingredients, plan meals effectively, and keep cooking essentials fresh.

CHAPTER 3
THE SCIENCE OF NUTRIENT-RICH COOKING

"The Science of Cooking Nutrient-Dense Foods in the Healthy Kitchen: Enjoying Good Health"

At Wellness Kitchen, the art of cooking and the science of nutrition are intertwined, creating a harmonious symphony that promotes optimal health. Understanding the science of cooking nutrient-dense foods is essential to creating dishes that not only excite the taste buds but also nourish the body.

1. **Methods of preserving nutrients**

Explore techniques like steaming, frying, and baking to preserve the maximum nutritional value of ingredients. These methods help preserve vitamins and minerals, ensuring that your meals are a source of essential nutrients.

2. **Smart combination of ingredients**

Discover the secrets of strategic ingredient combinations. Combining certain foods improves nutrient absorption, allowing the body to make the most of the available vitamins and minerals. Learn how to create synergistic combinations for a complete meal.

3. **The effect of cooking methods on nutrients**

Identify the effects of different cooking methods on the nutritional value of foods. Understanding how heat, time, and cooking environment affect nutrients will allow you to make informed choices, and optimize the health benefits of your culinary creations.

4. **Adopt whole foods**

Emphasize eating whole, unprocessed foods. These nutrients contain a range of vitamins, minerals, and antioxidants that promote overall health. Discover the art of incorporating a variety of whole foods into your recipes.

5. **Conscious cooking for health**

Developing mindfulness in the kitchen while preparing food. Learn about the relationship between your cooking methods and nutritional results. Not only does thoughtful cooking improve the taste, but it also ensures that nutrients are retained to benefit your body.

6. **Macronutrient Balance**

Learn the importance of a balanced approach to macronutrients - protein, fat, and carbohydrates. Striking the right balance supports energy levels, muscle function, and overall metabolic health. Explore recipes that balance macronutrients.

7. Seasonal and local ingredients

Learn about the benefits of using seasonal and local ingredients. Freshness and ripeness help improve nutrient levels. Understanding the availability of seasonal ingredients allows you to create diverse, nutrient-rich menus.

8. Adapt to dietary preferences

Design nutrient-dense cooking to suit a variety of dietary preferences, whether vegetarian, vegan, paleo, or more. Learn how to meet specific dietary needs while accommodating different dietary preferences so everyone can enjoy good health at the Wellness Kitchen.

By understanding the science behind cooking nutrient-dense foods, you'll embark on a culinary journey that not only enriches your dining experience but also lays the foundation for long-term health. Being healthy becomes an art form, a delicious blend of flavors and nutrients in every carefully prepared dish.

UNDERSTANDING NUTRIENTS AND THEIR BENEFITS

Nutrients are the building blocks that nourish our bodies, promoting overall health and vitality.

1. Macronutrients
   - *Proteins*: Support muscle recovery and immune function.
   - *Carbohydrates*: Provide energy for daily activities.
   - *Fats* are essential for brain health and hormone production.

2. Micronutrients
   - *Vitamins*: They contribute to a variety of body functions, from immune support (vitamin C) to bone health (vitamin D).
   - *Minerals*: Play a critical role in enzyme function and maintaining proper fluid balance.

3. Fiber
   - It promotes digestion and helps maintain a healthy weight by promoting a feeling of fullness.

4. Antioxidants
   - Found in fruits and vegetables, they fight oxidative stress and support cellular health.

5. **Moisturizer**

Water is essential for nutrient absorption, temperature regulation, and general body functions.

6. **All Products**

Prioritizing complete, unprocessed foods guarantees a diverse nutrient intake.

ADVANTAGES OF A DIET HIGH IN NUTRIENTS

1. **More energy**

A healthy diet boosts vitality and lowers exhaustion.

2. **Immune Support**

Zinc and vitamin C are among the nutrients that fortify the immune system.

3. **Weight Management**

Eating a healthy, balanced diet aids in keeping your weight in check.

4. **Mental Health**

Omega-3 fatty acids promote stable moods and good brain function.

GUIDES FOR A KITCHEN CENTERED ON NUTRIENTS

1. **Vibrant Plate**

This plate has an array of vibrant, nutrient-dense fruits and vegetables.

2. **Lean Proteins**

Select proteins from lean sources including fish, poultry, and plants.

3. **Whole Grains**

To obtain more fiber and nutrients, choose whole grains rather than refined grains.

By understanding the role of nutrients and incorporating them into your culinary choices, the wellness kitchen becomes a haven for savoring good health, fostering a balanced and nourished lifestyle.

COOKING METHODS TO PRESERVE NUTRITIONAL VALUE

At The Wellness Kitchen, preserving food's nutritious worth is crucial to fostering wellness. The following cooking techniques can aid in the preservation of nutrients:

1. **Cooking by Steam**

Using steam to prepare food minimizes nutrient loss during this mild cooking process. Steaming vegetables helps retain water-soluble vitamins like C, which makes them extremely healthy.

2. **Searing**

The nutrients in the vegetables are preserved when they are stir-fried at a reasonable temperature with a small amount of oil. This is an excellent method for protecting heat-sensitive vitamins and minerals.

3. **Searing and Charcoal**

The best cooking techniques for retaining the nutrients in meats and vegetables are those that use dry heat. Cook for moderate amounts of time to avoid losing too many nutrients, and use pickles to enhance flavor without compromising nutritional value

4. **Microwaving**

Contrary to popular belief, using a microwave for cooking can save the environment. It reduces nutrient leaching because it is quick and consumes little water. Avoid overcooking, nevertheless, to preserve the highest possible nutritious content.

5. **Vegetables Without** Fillers

Vegetables retain color, texture, and nutritional value when briefly boiled in boiling water and then swiftly cooled. Green beans and broccoli are two veggies that benefit greatly from this technique.

6. **Unprocessed or slightly altered**

The best way to retain nutrients in fruits and vegetables is to eat them raw or with little processing. If you're concerned about your health, think about including salads, smoothies, or raw snacks in your diet.

7. **Reduced Heating**

Slow cooking at lower temperatures can help preserve nutrients even though it takes longer to cook. This is a very good way to chop meat and flavorful veggies and lentils.

8. **Pressurized Cooking**

When compared to boiling or sautéing, pressure cooking helps preserve more vitamins and minerals while cutting down on cooking time. It works well with beans, cereals, and vegetables that are high in starch.

Recall that the secret to preparing delectable, fulfilling meals at The Wellness Kitchen is striking a balance between maintaining nutrients. By following these tips, you can enhance not just the flavor of your food but also your general health and well-being.

CHAPTER 4
MINDFUL EATING: THE FOUNDATION OF WELLNESS

In the hustle and bustle of our daily lives, eating often becomes a chore, overwhelmed by the demands of our schedule. However, mindful eating can be a transformative step toward overall health.

Mindful eating is more than just paying attention to what's on your plate; It's about developing a deep awareness of the entire eating process. Here are the basic principles to help you stay healthy at The Wellness Kitchen:

1. **Present Moment Awareness**
   Fully engage your senses while eating. Appreciate the colors, textures, and aromas of your food. By being fully present, you create a deeper connection with food.

2. **Enjoy every bite**
   Take time to savor every sip. Chew slowly, allowing your body to become familiar with the taste and texture. This not only improves digestion but also enhances feelings of satisfaction.

3. **Listen to your body**

Listen to your body's signals about hunger and fullness. Mindful eating involves understanding when you're truly hungry and recognizing when you're full, which prevents overeating.

4. Gratitude for food

Cultivate gratitude for the food on your plate. Recognize the effort and resources that go into preparing your food. This practice promotes a positive relationship with food and a sense of abundance.

5. Eliminate distractions

Minimize distractions while eating. Turn off screens, put away electronic devices, and create a quiet environment. This allows you to focus on the process of eating, promoting a conscious connection with food.

6. Listen to your body

Pay attention to the way different foods make you feel. Pay attention to the effect on your energy levels, mood, and general well-being. This awareness can help you make choices that fit your body's needs.

7. Intuitive Eating

Trust your body's signals and desires. Intuitive eating involves listening to your body's natural hunger cues and choosing foods that truly meet your nutritional needs.

By incorporating these principles into your daily routine, mindful eating will become the foundation of your health journey. It is a powerful tool that not only supports physical health but also promotes a harmonious relationship between your body and the nutrition it receives. At The Wellness Kitchen, being healthy starts with taking every bite with care, creating a path to holistic wellness.

THE ART OF MINDFUL EATING

In the world of mindful eating, every bite becomes a symphony of sensations—a harmonious dance of flavors, textures, and nutrients. The art of mindful eating goes beyond simple consumption; It is a practice that invites us to savor every bite and develop a deep connection with food.

At the art of mindful eating is awareness of the present moment. In the frantic pace of modern life, nutrition often takes a backseat to the fast pace of our schedules. However, mindfulness in a healthy kitchen allows us to break out of this vicious cycle. When we sit down to eat, we fully engage our senses, from the vibrant colors on the plate to the aromas in the air.

One of the key aspects of mindful eating is listening to our body's signals. Instead of eating automatically, we learn to recognize hunger and fullness, allowing our body to guide us. This intuitive approach promotes a balanced relationship with food, which promotes not only physical health but also emotional well-being.

Mindful eating goes beyond the plate and includes where our food comes from. By appreciating the journey from farm to table, we develop gratitude for the food the land provides. This connection to source improves our overall sense of well-being, creating a ripple effect that resonates with the choices we make in the wellness kitchen.

In the bustling world of The Wellness Kitchen, the art of mindful eating invites us to slow down and savor the sensory experience of every bite. Through this intentional practice, we not only enjoy good health, but we also rediscover the joy inherent in the simple act of nourishing our bodies.

BUILDING HEALTHY EATING HABITS

In the pursuit of well-being, developing healthy eating habits is the cornerstone of living a balanced and fulfilling life. The Wellness Kitchen will be the heart of this journey and where the art of being healthy begins.

1. **Choose whole foods**

Start by embracing a vibrant array of whole foods. Fill your plate with plenty of fruits, vegetables, whole grains, and lean proteins. These nutrient-dense foods contain essential vitamins, minerals, and antioxidants to keep your body functioning optimally.

2. **Practice mindful eating**

Practice mindful eating to improve your connection with food. Engage your senses, savor every bite, and pay attention to your hunger and fullness cues. This approach promotes a deeper understanding of the nutrition your body receives and promotes a healthy relationship with food.

3. **Hydration is the key to success**

Maintain proper hydration by including plenty of water in your daily routine. Water supports digestion, nutrient absorption, and overall cellular function. Infuse your water with natural flavors like citrus or herbs to make hydration fun and tempting.

4. Part control

Focus on portion control to find a balance between enjoying your favorite foods and maintaining a healthy lifestyle. Pay attention to portion sizes and listen to your body's signals to avoid overeating. This conscious approach promotes weight control and maintaining sustainable energy levels.

5. Variety on your plate

Prepare varied and complete meals that include different food groups. It provides a wide range of nutrients that promote overall health. Experiment with different recipes and cuisines to keep your meals interesting and satisfying.

6. Planning and preparation

Set yourself up for success by planning and preparing your meals in advance. This reduces your reliance on processed and convenience foods, allowing you to make informed choices that align with your health goals. Set aside time for meal prep to simplify your daily routine.

7. Listen to your body

Learn about your body's unique needs. Pay attention to the way certain foods make you feel and adjust your choices accordingly. Creating a personalized approach to nutrition that supports your well-being, taking into account individual needs and preferences.

8. Incremental changes for long-term success

Make changes gradually to build lasting habits. Small, consistent adjustments to your lifestyle are more likely to take hold. Celebrate every success and view your journey toward healthy eating as an ongoing positive development.

At The Wellness Kitchen, building healthy eating habits is a continuous process of discovery and enjoyment. By enjoying the benefits of whole foods, practicing mindfulness, and making informed choices, you set the stage for a life of vitality and longevity.

CHAPTER 5
BREAKFASTS THAT FUEL YOUR DAY

Start Your Day Right with Energizing Breakfasts

In "The Wellness Kitchen: Savoring Good Health," we emphasize the importance of breakfasts that fuel your day. A nourishing morning meal not only jump starts your metabolism but also provides sustained energy, setting a positive tone for the day ahead.

1. **Power-Packed Protein Pancakes**
   Kick off your morning with a stack of protein-packed pancakes. Blend oats, eggs, and a scoop of your favorite protein powder for a delicious and satisfying breakfast that keeps you full and focused.

2. **Nutrient-Rich Smoothie Bowls**
   Blend a vibrant mix of fruits, leafy greens, and a protein source like Greek yogurt or nut butter. Top it with crunchy granola, seeds, and a drizzle of honey for a refreshing bowl that nourishes your body and mind.

3. **Hearty Quinoa Breakfast Bowl**
   Elevate your breakfast game with a quinoa bowl loaded with nutrient-dense toppings. Combine cooked quinoa with fresh berries, sliced almonds,

and a dollop of Greek yogurt for a wholesome and filling start to your day.

4. Egg-cellent Avocado Toast

Avocado toast is a timeless favorite, and for good reason. Top whole-grain toast with mashed avocado and a perfectly poached egg. The combination of healthy fats and protein will keep you satisfied until your next meal.

5. Overnight Oats with a Twist

Prepare a batch of overnight oats by soaking rolled oats in milk or yogurt overnight. Add your favorite toppings like sliced fruits, nuts, and a dash of cinnamon for a convenient and nutritious breakfast that requires minimal morning effort.

6. Homemade Breakfast Burritos

Roll up a nutritious burst of flavor with a homemade breakfast burrito. Fill a whole-grain tortilla with scrambled eggs, black beans, diced vegetables, and a sprinkle of cheese for a delicious and portable morning treat.

Remember, a well-balanced breakfast sets the foundation for a day filled with vitality and wellness. Experiment with these recipes and discover the joy of savoring good health from the very first meal.

ENERGIZING MORNING MEALS

Start your day with a burst of energy by choosing nutritious and delicious morning meals from The Wellness Kitchen: Savoring Good Health. Our energizing breakfast options are designed to fuel your body, kickstart your metabolism, and set a positive tone for the day ahead.

1. **Quinoa Power Bowl**
   - Packed with protein, fiber, and essential nutrients, our quinoa power bowl combines cooked quinoa with fresh berries, nuts, and a drizzle of honey. This wholesome breakfast will keep you feeling full and energized throughout the morning.

2. **Green Smoothie Delight**
   - Blend up a vibrant green smoothie using spinach, kale, banana, and a splash of almond milk. Rich in vitamins and antioxidants, this refreshing beverage not only nourishes your body but also contributes to a revitalized start to your day.

3. **Protein-Packed Oatmeal**
   - Upgrade your traditional oatmeal by adding a scoop of protein powder, sliced fruits, and a sprinkle of chia seeds. This hearty bowl not only provides sustained energy but also supports muscle

recovery, making it an ideal choice for an active morning.

4. Egg and Avocado Toast

- Enjoy a savory breakfast with whole-grain toast topped with mashed avocado and a perfectly poached egg. Packed with healthy fats and protein, this combination will keep you feeling satisfied and ready to tackle your daily tasks.

5. Chia Seed Pudding Parfait

- Indulge in a delightful chia seed pudding layered with Greek yogurt and fresh fruit. This meal not only satisfies your sweet cravings but also offers a good balance of macronutrients to keep you energized and focused.

At The Wellness Kitchen, we believe that a nourishing breakfast is the foundation of a day filled with vitality. Choose from our selection of energizing morning meals to support your well-being and savor the taste of good health every morning.

RECIPES FOR A NUTRIENT-PACKED BREAKFAST

Start your day on a nutritious note with these recipes for a nutrient-packed breakfast in the Wellness Kitchen. Fuel your body with wholesome ingredients that promote good health and sustained energy throughout the day.

1. Power-Packed Smoothie Bowl

Blend a mix of kale, spinach, banana, berries, and a scoop of protein powder for a vibrant and nutrient-rich smoothie bowl. Top it with nuts, seeds, and a drizzle of honey for added flavor and texture.

2. Quinoa Breakfast Bowl

Swap out traditional grains for quinoa, a protein-packed superfood. Cook it with almond milk and add sliced fruits, nuts, and a sprinkle of cinnamon for a delicious and hearty breakfast bowl that will keep you satisfied.

3. Avocado Toast with a Twist

Elevate your classic avocado toast by adding poached eggs, cherry tomatoes, and a sprinkle of chia seeds. This combination provides a good balance of healthy fats, protein, and essential vitamins.

4. **Chia Seed Pudding Parfait**

Combine chia seeds with almond milk and let them soak overnight. In the morning, layer the pudding with Greek yogurt, fresh fruits, and a drizzle of agave nectar. This parfait is rich in omega-3 fatty acids and antioxidants.

5. **Egg White Vegetable Omelet**

Whisk together egg whites and sauté them with a colorful array of vegetables like bell peppers, spinach, and tomatoes. Packed with protein and vitamins, this omelet is a savory and satisfying breakfast option.

6. **Homemade Granola with Yogurt**

Create your granola using oats, nuts, seeds, and a touch of honey. Serve it over Greek yogurt and add sliced fruits for a crunchy and creamy breakfast that's high in fiber and beneficial probiotics.

7. **Sweet Potato and Black Bean Breakfast Burrito**

Wrap up a nutritious mix of sweet potatoes, black beans, scrambled eggs, and a sprinkle of cheese in a whole-grain tortilla. This savory breakfast burrito is a hearty and flavorful way to start your day.

Remember, a nutrient-packed breakfast sets the tone for a day filled with vitality and well-being.

Experiment with these recipes to discover your favorite combinations and embrace the joy of savoring good health in the Wellness Kitchen.

CHAPTER 6
SMART CHOICES FOR MIDDAY NUTRITION

In the frantic pace of our daily lives, making conscious midday meal choices is essential to maintaining overall health. The Wellness Kitchen encourages people to stay healthy by making smart nutrition decisions during those crucial midday hours. Here are some basic principles to help you prepare a nutritious and satisfying lunch:

1. Balanced Macronutrients
Make sure your afternoon snack is a harmonious combination of carbohydrates, proteins, and healthy fats. Choose whole grains, lean proteins such as poultry or legumes, and sources of unsaturated fats such as avocados or nuts to maintain energy levels throughout the day.

2. Colorful, Nutrient-Rich Vegetables
Liven up your afternoon snack by including a variety of colorful vegetables. These nutrient-rich powerhouses not only add flavor and texture, but also provide essential vitamins, minerals, and antioxidants needed to maintain good health.

3. Precise Portion Control
Practice portion control to prevent overeating and improve digestion. Pay attention to your hunger

cues and consciously savor each bite. Eating well-portioned meals helps maintain energy levels without causing sluggishness.

4. Hydration Habits

Stay hydrated by including water-rich foods such as fruits and vegetables in your midday menu. Proper hydration supports digestion, improves cognitive function, and helps regulate body temperature.

5. Whole Foods vs. Processed Foods

Choose whole, unprocessed foods instead of their processed counterparts. Whole foods are rich in nutrients and fiber, which promotes better digestion and provides a steady release of energy, keeping you energized throughout the rest of the day.

6. Mindful Eating

Develop the habit of mindful eating by sitting down and enjoying your midday meal without distractions. This practice improves the taste of food by allowing you to savor flavors and recognize satiety cues, leading to more satisfying, healthier meals.

7. Individual dietary needs

Recognize and meet your individual nutritional needs. When planning your midday feeding, consider dietary preferences, allergies, and specific health goals. Personalizing your selection ensures you have food that suits your unique luxury travel experience.

By eating these smart midday meal options, you'll not only nourish your body, but you'll also contribute to The Wellness Kitchen's ethos of wellness. Remember, every bite is an opportunity to invest in your well-being and enjoy the journey to a healthier, more vibrant life.

TASTY AND HEALTHY LUNCH IDEAS

Savoring health is not simply a motto, but a way of life at The Wellness Kitchen. Eating wholesome, delectable meals is crucial for maintaining general health. These are some delicious and health-conscious lunch options that will fuel your body and satisfy your taste senses.

1. Quinoa Salad Delight
 - Combine cooked quinoa, cucumber, feta cheese, cherry tomatoes, and colorful bell peppers.
 - Serve with a simple vinaigrette of lemon juice, olive oil, and a dash of herbs.
 - This salad, which is full of protein and antioxidants, makes a light and filling lunch choice.

2. Grilled Chicken Wraps
 - Place lean chicken strips between whole-grain tortillas and grill them.
  - Include a rainbow of vegetables, such as red cabbage, shredded carrots, and spinach.
  - Finish it with a tangy sauce made of yogurt for a low-carb, high-protein meal.

3. Mediterranean Power Bowl
 – Mix cucumber, cherry tomatoes, olives, cooked quinoa, or brown rice with chickpeas.

- For a bowl full of heart-healthy fats and fiber, take inspiration from the Mediterranean and add some extra virgin olive oil and feta cheese.

4. Tofu with Vegetables Stir-Fried
 - Sauté bell peppers, broccoli, snap peas, and other colorful veggies with tofu cubes.
 - Add some ginger, garlic, and low-sodium soy sauce to make it a pleasant, nutrient- and protein-rich plant-based lunch alternative.

5. Salmon and Avocado Sushi Bowls
 - Assemble cooked salmon, sliced avocado, seaweed strips, and brown rice into deconstructed sushi bowls.
 - For a lunch that's high in nutrients and omega-3 fatty acids, drizzle with a mild soy sauce and top with sesame seeds.

6. Brahma Bowl with Sweet Potato and Chickpeas
 - Roast chickpeas and sweet potato cubes using a spice mixture that includes paprika and cumin.
- Put them in a bowl with avocado slices, fresh greens, and tahini dressing for a filling and healthy lunch alternative.

The Wellness Kitchen offers a variety of delicious and healthful lunch alternatives that are sure to please your palate and nourish your body. Try out these recipes to find the ideal ratio of nutrients to flavor, which will make your path to better health enjoyable.

CHAPTER 7
WHOLESOME DINNERS FOR OPTIMAL WELL-BEING

In The Wellness Kitchen: Enjoying Wellness, we explore the art of preparing healthy meals that nourish the body and promote overall well-being. These carefully selected recipes prioritize nutritional balance, flavor, and cooking pleasure to promote a healthy lifestyle.

1. **Quinoa Power Bowl**
   - Protein quinoa base with a vibrant medley of roasted vegetables.

   Garnish with avocado slices, a pinch of seeds, and a little olive oil to get more essential nutrients.

2. **Salmon and citrus salad**
   - Grilled salmon filet with citrus orange and grapefruit salad.

   The omega-3 fatty acids in salmon promote heart health, and the citrus fruits provide a refreshing taste.

3. **Lentil-vegetable stew**
   - Delicious stew with fiber-rich lentils and a variety of flavorful vegetables, herbs, and spices.

Rich in plant-based proteins, vitamins, and minerals, this soup supports digestive health and provides consistent energy.

4. Sweet Potato and Chickpea Curry

- Creamy sweet potato and chickpea curry cooked in an aromatic spice blend.

This dish is a powerful source of antioxidants, fiber, and anti-inflammatory properties.

5. Grilled chicken with quinoa salad

- Grilled chicken breasts served with quinoa salad stuffed with fresh herbs, tomatoes, and cucumbers.

High-quality chicken protein combined with the nutritional value of quinoa makes this a filling and satisfying dinner.

6. Stuffed Mediterranean Peppers

- Stuffed bell peppers with a mixture of ground turkey, quinoa, tomatoes, and Mediterranean herbs.

Rich in antioxidants and lean protein, this dish reflects the heart-healthy aspects of the Mediterranean diet.

7. Fried with vegetables

- A colorful stir-fry with a variety of crunchy vegetables and tofu or lean beef.

- This dish is quick to prepare and ensures a variety of vitamins and minerals for overall health.

8. Zucchini noodles with pesto sauce and cherry tomatoes

Spiral zucchini noodles with bright basil pesto and cherry tomatoes.

- A low-carb option that combines the taste of summer while providing essential nutrients.

At the Health Kitchen, these recipes not only excite the palate but also empower people to make informed, health-oriented choices in their culinary endeavors. Each dish invites you to savor the flavors of whole, unprocessed ingredients, promoting optimal well-being and a deep awareness of the connection between food and vitality.

CREATING BALANCED DINNER PLATES

At The Wellness Kitchen, achieving and maintaining good health is not just about what you eat, but also how you balance your plate. A balanced plate not only stimulates the taste buds, but also provides a symphony of nutrients that your body needs. Here's a guide to making plates that balance flavor and health.

1. **Multicolored canvas**

Colorful vegetables should dominate your plate. Aim for a rainbow of colors, as each shade contains a unique array of vitamins, minerals and antioxidants. Include leafy greens, peppers, carrots and other seasonal vegetables to create a visually appealing and nutritious base.

2. **The Power of Protein**

A well-balanced plate contains lean protein. Whether it's grilled chicken, fish, tofu or legumes, protein plays a critical role in muscle recovery, immune function and overall satiety. Choose a variety of protein sources to provide a spectrum of essential amino acids.

3. **Healthy grains**

Good carbohydrates are essential for maintaining stable energy levels. Choose whole grains such as quinoa, brown rice or whole wheat pasta. They contain complex carbohydrates, fiber, and essential nutrients that support digestive health and keep you feeling full and satisfied.

4. Healthy fats

Don't avoid fats; just choose wisely. Include healthy sources of fats in your diet, such as avocados, nuts, seeds and olive oil. These fats are essential for nutrient absorption, brain function, and healthy skin.

5. Dairy products or dairy substitutes

Calcium is critical for bone health, so include fortified dairy products or dairy substitutes such as almond or soy milk in your diet. Greek yogurt is a great choice because it contains protein and probiotics for gut health.

6. Be mindful of portions

Practice portion control to avoid overeating. Use smaller plates and listen to your body's hunger and satiety signals. This simple habit can make a big difference in weight management and overall well-being.

7. Harmonious hydration

Complete your balanced diet with a glass of water. Staying hydrated is vital for digestion, nutrient absorption, and overall body function. Consider adding fresh herbs or fruit to your water for added flavor without added sugar.

At The Wellness Kitchen, preparing balanced plates is a celebration of health, taste and mindful eating. By including a variety of colorful, nutrient-dense foods in your diet, you're not just enjoying delicious food: you're nourishing your body for optimal well-being.

DINNER RECIPES TO BOOST YOUR HEALTH

In a world where health takes center stage, the importance of nourishing your body with healthy foods cannot be overstated. Transform your table into a health oasis with these delicious recipes designed to improve your well-being.

1. Quinoa and Vegetable Stir-Fry
   - Quinoa, packed with protein and fiber, forms the basis of this nutrient-rich stir-fry. Combine colorful vegetables such as peppers, broccoli, and carrots for a boost of vitamins and antioxidants. Top with a light sesame ginger sauce for added flavor and health benefits.

2. Salmon with Lemon-Dill Sauce
   - Rich in omega-3 fatty acids, salmon is good for your heart. Bake or grill salmon filets and top them with a tangy lemon-dill sauce. This not only improves the taste but also adds a dose of antioxidants that support cardiovascular and immune health.

3. Mediterranean Chickpea Salad
   - Adopt a Mediterranean diet with a refreshing chickpea salad. Combine chickpeas with cherry tomatoes, cucumbers, olives, and feta cheese. Add

olive oil and herbs for a dish that is not only delicious but also promotes digestive health and satiety.

4. Sweet Potato and Black Bean Enchiladas

- Replace traditional enchiladas with healthier options made with sweet potatoes and black beans. These ingredients contain complex carbohydrates and protein, as well as fiber. Top with bright tomato salsa for an extra vitamin boost.

5. Spinach and Mushroom Quiche with Whole Wheat Crust

- Top off your dinner with nutrient-rich quiche. Use a whole wheat crust to add fiber and fill it with a mixture of spinach, mushrooms, and eggs. This dish is rich in iron, vitamins, and protein, which promote overall energy and immune support.

6. Kebab of grilled chicken and vegetables

- Prepare a simple and tasty dish with grilled chicken and vegetable kebabs. Marinate chicken pieces in a light citrus marinade and thread them onto skewers with colorful peppers, zucchini, and cherry tomatoes. The combination provides a balanced mixture of proteins and vitamins.

7. Cauliflower Fried Rice

- Give your favorite classic dish a twist by replacing rice with cauliflower. Packed with veggies, eggs, and a little soy sauce, this low-carb alternative is perfect for those looking for a lighter option without sacrificing flavor.

Dinner isn't just about food; This is an opportunity to saturate the body with essential nutrients. Include these recipes in The Wellness Kitchen and enjoy the benefits that promote physical and mental well-being.

CHAPTER 8
SAVORING GOOD HEALTH WITH SWEETS

Eating sweets can be a delicious way to stay healthy if done mindfully. Choosing naturally sweet treats, like those rich in fruit, or using alternatives like honey and maple syrup, not only adds sweetness but also nutritional value. This choice provides antioxidants, vitamins, and minerals that promote general well-being.

Including dark chocolate in your diet is another healthy strategy. Dark chocolate is known for its flavonoid content, which has been linked to heart health and improved cognitive function. Choose options with a higher cocoa content for maximum benefits.

Balancing sweet cravings with nutritious ingredients like whole grains and nuts can turn desserts into a constant source of energy. Experimenting with recipes that include oat, quinoa, or almond flour will give a healthy twist to traditional treats.

Remember that enjoying sweets for health means consuming them in moderation and appreciating the natural benefits they provide. Whether it's a fruit dessert, a bar of dark chocolate, or a treat made with nutrient-rich ingredients, the key to mindful eating is balancing pleasure and well-being.

GUILT-FREE DESSERT OPTIONS

At The Wellness Kitchen, committing to a healthy lifestyle doesn't mean sacrificing the joy of delicious desserts. Discover guilt-free alternatives that will not only satisfy your sweet tooth but also support your overall well-being. These dessert options prioritize nutrient-rich ingredients for a delicious balance of flavor and health.

1. **Avocado mousse with dark chocolate**

Immerse yourself in the velvety richness of a chocolate mousse that captures all the goodness of an avocado. Packed with heart-healthy fats and antioxidants, this guilt-free treat is sure to please your taste buds without compromising your health.

2. **Chia seed pudding parfait**

Switch up your dessert with this chia seed pudding parfait. Filled with fresh fruit and low-fat yogurt, this delicious creation is a fantastic source of omega-3 fatty acids, fiber, and essential nutrients.

3. **Baked Apple Delight**

Feel the soothing warmth of baked apples lightly sweetened with natural honey or maple syrup. This simple but satisfying dessert option is rich in fiber and vitamins, making it the perfect choice for an enjoyable evening.

4. Frozen banana pieces

Savor the sweetness of frozen banana pieces coated in a thin layer of dark chocolate. Not only do they provide a natural energy boost, but they also contain potassium and magnesium, which support heart health and muscle function.

5. Greek Yogurt Berry parfait

Indulge in the bright colors and flavors of this berry Greek yogurt parfait. Packed with antioxidants, vitamins, and probiotics, this dessert not only satisfies your sweet tooth but also promotes gut health.

6. Chocolate Quinoa Crispy Bars

Up your dessert game with these crunchy chocolate quinoa bars. These nutrient-rich treats combine the goodness of quinoa, nuts, and dark chocolate, delivering a satisfying crunch and delivering a dose of essential minerals and antioxidants.

At The Wellness Kitchen, enjoying good health doesn't mean saying goodbye to dessert. These guilt-free options will allow you to enjoy the good life while nourishing your body with healthy ingredients. Enjoy these delicious alternatives and

turn every dessert into a celebration of wellness at
The Wellness Kitchen.

HEALTHY DESSERT RECIPES TO SATISFY YOUR SWEET TOOTH

You may still maintain your dedication to a healthy lifestyle while indulging in sweets. Find a mouthwatering assortment of guilt-free sweets that can satiate your desires and enhance your general health. The Wellness Kitchen provides a selection of recipes that put health and flavor first, from nutrient-rich smoothies to nutritious fruit snacks.

1. **Parfait with chia seeds**

Start with a parfait of chia seed pudding to begin your delicious adventure. After combining the chia seeds and almond milk, refrigerate overnight. For a filling and healthy treat, sprinkle chopped nuts and fresh berries over the custard.

2. **Boiled banana chunks**

For an easy yet opulent treat, freeze banana slices and dip them in dark chocolate. Antioxidants are found in dark chocolate, and frozen bananas have a creamy texture. Add shredded coconut or chopped nuts for further flavor.

3. **Hairspray Smoothie with Berries**

For a vibrant and reviving smoothie, combine berries and Greek yogurt together. For a lovely crunch and natural sweetness, sprinkle some granola, sliced almonds, and honey on top.

4. Mousse with avocado and chocolate

Try this avocado and chocolate mousse instead of the standard one. Blend the mature avocados with the cacao powder and add maple syrup for sweetness. This creamy, silky dessert is packed full of antioxidants and good fats.

5. Raisin and Oatmeal Energy Snacks

For a quick energy boost, combine muesli, raisins and a small pinch of cinnamon. For a quick and healthy snack that will satisfy your sweet appetite without adding extra sugar, these no-bake snacks are ideal.

6. Popsicles and yogurt

To make your popsicles, combine pureed fresh fruit with Greek yogurt. These vibrant candies are a great source of vitamins and probiotics in addition to being aesthetically pleasing.

7. Baked Apple with Cinnamon

Enjoy the pure flavor of baked apples with a honey drizzle and cinnamon sprinkling. This warm, soothing dessert is the ideal guilt-free treat because it's strong in fiber and low in calories.

Experience the delight of crafting desserts at The Wellness Kitchen that prioritize your well-being without sacrificing flavor. These recipes show that indulging your sweet appetite can be a tasty, healthful pastime that enhances general wellbeing.

CHAPTER 9
WELLNESS KITCHEN MEAL PLANS

A variety of meal plans are available from The Wellness Kitchen: Savouring Good Health, which is intended to support general wellbeing. These carefully chosen diets put an emphasis on wholesome, whole foods to nourish your body and encourage a healthy way of living.

1. Nutrients in Balance
A balanced combination of vital elements, such as proteins, carbs, healthy fats, vitamins, and minerals, is the main goal of our meal plans. This guarantees that your body gets the nourishment it requires to function at its best.

2. Fresh and Seasonal Ingredients
To optimize flavor and nutritional value, we place a strong emphasis on using fresh, in-season ingredients. Our meal plans offer a range of health advantages and diversity to keep your palette satisfied.

3. Tailoring to Dietary Requirements
The Wellness Kitchen creates meal plans that are customized to your nutritional needs, whether you're a vegetarian, vegan, gluten-free, or follow another diet. Since we think that everyone's journey

to wellness is unique, our strategies take that into account.

4. Intentional Consumption

Not limited to the components, our meal plans promote mindful eating. You can cultivate a positive relationship with food by taking the time to appreciate every bite and paying attention to signals of hunger and fullness.

5. Control of Portion

A crucial component of our meal planning is portion control, which encourages balance and deters overindulgence. This method facilitates digestion and aids in maintaining a healthy weight.

6. Hydration Assistance

It's essential to stay hydrated for general wellness. To keep you energized and support numerous body functions, our meal plans include foods that are high in water content and encourage you to drink plenty of it.

7. Easy Meal Preparation

The Wellness Kitchen is aware of the pressures of contemporary living. Our meal plans include doable and realistic meal prep techniques, so it's easy for you to maintain your wellness objectives.

8. Learning Materials

We offer instructional materials on nutrition, cooking methods, and the advantages of particular items in addition to meal ideas. Providing you with information is a vital component of our dedication to your welfare.

Start your path to wellness by utilizing The Wellness Kitchen. Savor the goodness of hearty, delectable meals that feed your mind and spirit.

WEEKLY MEAL PLANS FOR BALANCED NUTRITION

In The Wellness Kitchen, we believe that good health starts with nourishing your body with a well-balanced diet. Our weekly meal plans are designed to not only tantalize your taste buds but also provide the essential nutrients your body needs for optimal health. Here's a glimpse into a week of flavorful and nutritious meals:

Day 1: Energizing Monday

- *Breakfast*: Quinoa and Berry Parfait
- *Lunch:* Grilled Chicken Salad with a variety of colorful vegetables
- *Dinner*: Baked Salmon with Roasted Sweet Potatoes and Steamed Broccoli

Day 2: Meatless Tuesday

- *Breakfast*: Spinach and Feta Omelette
- *Lunch*: Lentil and Vegetable Stir-Fry
- *Dinner*: Stuffed Bell Peppers with Quinoa and Black Beans

Day 3: Wholesome Wednesday

- *Breakfast*: Overnight Oats with Chia Seeds and Mixed Berries
- *Lunch*: Turkey and Avocado Wrap with Whole Grain Tortilla
- *Dinner:* Baked Cod with Lemon Herb Quinoa and Sautéed Spinach

Day 4: Plant-Powered Thursday

- *Breakfast*: Banana Walnut Smoothie with Greek Yogurt
- *Lunch:* Chickpea and Vegetable Curry
- *Dinner:* Grilled Portobello Mushrooms with Brown Rice and Asparagus

Day 5: Fiesta Friday

- *Breakfast*: Huevos Rancheros with Salsa
- *Lunch*: Shrimp and Black Bean Salad
- *Dinner:* Chicken Fajita Bowl with Quinoa and Peppers

Day 6: Satisfying Saturday

- *Breakfast*: Whole Grain Pancakes with Fresh Fruit
- *Lunch*: Quinoa and Vegetable Buddha Bowl
- *Dinner*: Beef and Vegetable Stir-Fry with Brown Rice

Day 7: Relaxing Sunday

- *Breakfast*: Greek Yogurt Parfait with Nuts and Honey
- *Lunch*: Caprese Salad with Grilled Chicken
- *Dinner*: Roasted Vegetable and Chickpea Stew

Remember to stay hydrated throughout the week by incorporating water, herbal teas, and infused water into your routine. These meal plans are crafted not only for delicious dining but also to support your overall well-being. Embrace The Wellness Kitchen's approach to savoring good health through a variety of nutrient-packed, flavorful meals. Cheers to a week of balanced nutrition and vitality!

CUSTOMIZING MEAL PLANS FOR YOUR NEEDS

In The Wellness Kitchen, a personalized meal plan is a key step towards good health. Tailoring dishes to your specific needs not only improves taste but also optimizes nutrition. Here's a guide to customizing your meal plan to suit your individual needs:

1. Evaluate your dietary goals

Start by defining your health goals. Whether it's weight control, muscle gain, or dietary restrictions, understanding your goals forms the basis of a personalized nutrition plan.

2. Consider your nutritional needs

Assess your nutritional needs based on factors such as age, gender, activity level, and any existing health conditions. Ensure a balanced intake of proteins, carbohydrates, fats, vitamins, and minerals.

3. Explore your culinary preferences

Personalize your meals to include foods you love. Experiment with a variety of recipes according to your taste and make your journey to good health an enjoyable one.

4. **Portion control**

Choose portions based on your energy expenditure and weight goals. Moderation is key; Balance your plate with appropriately sized portions of proteins, grains, and vegetables.

5. **Adapt to dietary restrictions**

If you have dietary restrictions or allergies, adjust your meal plan accordingly. Change ingredients to suit your needs without sacrificing taste or nutrition.

6. **Meal frequency and time**

Customize your meal schedule based on your daily routine and preferences. Whether you prefer a few small meals or a few larger ones, find a rhythm that fits your lifestyle.

7. **Hydration is vital**

Do not forget about hydration. Personalize your beverage choices by including plenty of water, herbal teas, or other low-calorie beverages to support your overall well-being.

8. **Variety is the spice of life**

Make sure your eating plan includes a variety of foods that provide a wide range of nutrients. Not only does it increase your nutrient intake, but it also makes your meals interesting.

9. Monitoring and adjusting

Regularly evaluate how your body responds to your personalized nutritional plan. Adjustments may be necessary as your goals or lifestyle evolve.

10. Consult a nutritionist

For a more personalized approach, consult a nutritionist or nutritionist. They can provide expert advice tailored to your specific health needs.

Remember that the path to good health is unique to each person. By customizing your meal plan at The Wellness Kitchen, you're not only nourishing your body; you enjoy the path to well-being.

CHAPTER 10
DINING OUT AND SOCIAL WELLNESS

In our busy lives, eating out has become more than just a way to make ends meet; It has become a social experience that greatly affects our overall well-being. The Wellness Kitchen celebrates the synergy between eating out and social well-being, recognizing the deep connection between food, connection, and our mental and emotional well-being.

1. Body Nutrition

Eating out allows you to enjoy nutritious meals prepared with care. Wellness Kitchen emphasizes the importance of choosing restaurants that favor fresh, whole ingredients and a healthy, balanced diet. By making conscious choices when eating out, people can nourish their bodies and maintain their overall health.

2. Developing social connections

Sharing a meal goes beyond eating; it reinforces social ties and develops a sense of community. Wellness Kitchen encourages people to have dinner with friends, family, or colleagues, recognizing that these shared experiences foster diverse social bonds. Positive communication around the table improves our mental and emotional well-being.

3. **Mindful eating**

Wellness Kitchen promotes mindful eating and encourages people to enjoy every bite and have meaningful conversations while eating. By being present during a meal, people can connect more deeply with the food and the company they keep, resulting in a fulfilling and rewarding culinary journey.

4. **Various culinary discoveries**

Knowing different cuisines promotes an understanding of different cultures and tastes. At the Wellness Kitchen, we believe that different culinary experiences add enjoyment to our meals, but also broaden our understanding of global wellness practices. Eating out becomes a cultural journey that promotes a holistic approach to health.

5. **Balance between pleasure and health**

While delicious food is an integral part of dining out, the Wellness Kitchen emphasizes the importance of finding balance. By making conscious choices and choosing healthier options from time to time, people can enjoy eating without compromising their health goals.

Together, The Wellness Kitchen celebrates the intersection of dining out and social wellness, recognizing the profound impact these experiences have on our overall health. By making informed choices, strengthening social connections, and participating in various culinary adventures, people can enjoy a holistic approach to wellness beyond good food.

MAKING HEALTHY CHOICES AT RESTAURANTS

In a world where eating out is a shared pleasure, making healthy choices at restaurants is key to maintaining overall well-being. Holy Kitchen: Enjoy good health and encourage you to enjoy your dining experience by putting your health first. Here's a guide to help you make informed choices when browsing the menu.

1. **Start with water**

Start your meal with a glass of water. Not only will it keep you hydrated, but it can also help control your appetite and prevent you from overindulging.

2. **Explore the Menu**

Explore the menu thoroughly. Look for keywords like roasted, steamed, fried, or deep-fried, which are related to healthier cooking methods. Choose foods rich in lean protein, whole grains, and a variety of colorful vegetables.

3. **Portion Control**

Restaurants often serve larger portions than necessary. To avoid overeating, consider sharing an entree or asking for a half portion. Alternatively, you can ask for it at the start of the meal so you can save half for later.

4. **Note Changes**

Please change your order. Ask for side dishes and sauces, opt for steamed or stir-fried vegetables instead of fried options, and if possible whole grains or brown rice.

5. **Lean Protein Choices**

Choose lean protein sources such as grilled chicken, fish, or vegetables. These options provide essential nutrients without the added saturated fat typically found in fried or highly processed meats.

6. **Colorful plate**

Aim for a vibrant and versatile plate. Add a variety of colorful vegetables to ensure a diverse selection of vitamins and minerals. The more colors, the more nutritional value!

7. **Smart sides**

Instead of choosing fries or other fried sides, choose a side salad, steamed vegetables, or a small portion of a whole grain side dish to add fiber.

8. **Be careful with the sauce**

Dressings and sauces can add unnecessary calories. Request them on the page so you can check how much you're using. Consider using olive oil, lemon, or vinegar to add flavor without adding extra calories.

9. Balanced Choices

Aim for a balanced meal that includes a mix of carbohydrates, protein, and healthy fats. It not only satisfies your taste buds but also gives you constant energy.

10. Dessert Decisions

If you have a sweet tooth, share a dessert or go for a fruit-based option. Alternatively, enjoying a small portion of a decadent treat can be a great way to end a meal without overindulging. By following these conscious practices, you can enjoy eating out while putting your health first and Enjoy good health and believe that making informed choices in restaurants is a key ingredient in the recipe for overall well-being.

NAVIGATING SOCIAL SITUATIONS WHILE PRIORITIZING HEALTH

In today's busy world, maintaining a healthy lifestyle is essential, but it can be difficult in different social situations. The key is to find a balance between enjoying social interaction and prioritizing your health. Here are some tips for navigating social situations while enjoying good health:

1. **Conscious choices in meetings**

Be aware of your food and beverage choices at social events. Choose nutritious options and limit alcohol consumption. By combining indulgence and healthier choices, you can enjoy the moment without compromising your well-being.

2. **Tell us about your health goals**

Share your health goals with friends and family. Open communication helps set expectations and gain support. Whether it's choosing a restaurant with a healthier option or suggesting alternative activities, your loved ones can play an important role in fostering a health-conscious social environment.

3. **Be active together**

Instead of sedentary meetings, suggest activities that involve movement. Whether it's a walk in nature, a group workout, or even a night of dancing, combining physical activity with socializing can be both enjoyable and healthy.

4. Prioritize sleep

Sufficient sleep is the basis of good health. Kindly limit late events and prioritize adequate rest. Your well-being should come first, and your friends who understand your commitment to health will appreciate your honesty.

5. Hydration is key

Always stay hydrated, especially in social situations. Water not only supports your overall health, it can help you make informed choices about food and alcohol consumption. Bring a reusable water bottle so you have hydration readily available.

6. Plan Ahead

You anticipate social events and plan accordingly. Eat a nutritious meal before attending so you're less likely to snack on unhealthy snacks. Bringing a healthy portion to share at get-togethers ensures it's an option that aligns with your health priorities.

7. Practice moderation

While enjoying social events is important, moderation is key. Enjoy your favorite sweets now and then, but watch portions. This approach allows you to enjoy the moment without derailing your health journey.

Remember that navigating social situations while prioritizing health means finding a sustainable balance. By making informed choices, communicating effectively, and incorporating healthy habits into your social life, you can enjoy good health without losing the joy of connecting with others.

CHAPTER 11
WELLNESS COOKING FOR VEGETARIANS AND VEGANS

Healthy Cooking for Vegetarians and Vegans is a journey to nourish body, mind and soul with healthy plant-based ingredients. In the field of conscious cuisine, we celebrate the abundance of nature by creating culinary experiences where health is a priority without sacrificing taste.

Our recipes are vibrant colors and flavors derived from a variety of fruits, vegetables and vegetables. Rich in vitamins, minerals and antioxidants, these herbal ingredients form the basis of our wellness cuisine and promote overall health and vitality.

Protein takes center stage, with a focus on plant-based sources such as beans, lentils, chickpeas and tofu. These rich options not only promote muscle health, but also provide satisfying and sustainable protein levels that support an active and balanced lifestyle.

Whole grains, from quinoa to brown rice, become essential building blocks of our culinary creations. They are full of fiber, aid digestion and provide a constant release of energy, promoting a feeling of fullness and sustained vitality throughout the day.

The skill of seasoning in our wellness kitchen includes embracing herbs and spices for both their flavor-enhancing properties and potential health benefits. Turmeric, cumin and garlic not only enhance taste, but also contribute to anti-inflammatory and immune-boosting properties. At the heart of our approach are conscious cooking techniques that ensure the nutritional value of the ingredients is preserved. From steaming and boiling to roasting, each method is chosen to bring out the best in plant-based foods.

Beyond the plate, we encourage mindfulness in all aspects of the culinary journey. From conscious meal planning to purposeful enjoyment of every bite, wellness cooking becomes a holistic practice that reaches beyond the kitchen and fosters a deep connection between nutrition and well-being.

In our Vegetarian and Vegan Wellness Kitchen, we invite you to discover the joy of creating and enjoying meals that not only tempt your taste buds, but also boost your overall health and vitality. Take advantage of the richness of plant life, where well-being and culinary pleasure are intertwined in every delicious bite.

NUTRIENT-RICH COOKING FOR SPECIFIC DIETARY NEEDS

In The Wellness Kitchen: Hearing Good Health, we delve into the art of nutrient-dense cooking tailored to specific nutritional needs. Our culinary approach is not just about taste; it is the preparation of foods that promote well-being and vitality.

Understand Nutritional Needs

1. *Personalized nutrition*

See how to tailor meals to meet individual nutritional needs, taking into account factors such as age, gender, activity level, and health status.

2. *Special Diets*

Navigate a variety of diets, including gluten-free, dairy-free, vegetarian, and vegan, making sure every diet finds its place in your culinary repertoire.

Contains Nutrient-rich Ingredients

1. *Power Superfoods*

Learn how to add nutrient-dense superfoods like kale, quinoa, chia seeds, and berries to your cooking to boost the nutritional content of your meals.

2. *Balanced Macronutrients*

Learn how to balance protein, carbohydrates, and healthy fats to create varied, satisfying meals that support sustained energy levels.

Cooking Techniques For Maximum Food Preservation

1. *Steaming and Roasting*

Discover the benefits of steaming and roasting, preserving the vitamin and mineral integrity of ingredients and enhancing flavors for a healthy eating experience.

2. *Minimal Processing*

Master the art of minimal processing to preserve the nutritional value of fresh, whole foods and create foods that nourish the body without unnecessary additives.

Delicious And Functional Recipes

1. *Culinary Alchemy*

Explore innovative ways to add flavor to dishes with herbs, spices, and aromatics. Otherwise, every meal becomes a delightful experience that serves both taste buds and health purposes.

2. *Meal Planning*

Consider careful meal planning and make sure each plate is a symphony of colors, textures, and nutrients that promote overall well-being.

A Wellness Kitchen Experience

Embark on a journey where cooking is not just a daily chore, but a conscious effort to enjoy good health. The Wellness Kitchen invites you to transform your relationship with food, making every meal a celebration of nutrition, taste, and vitality.

Note. Always consult a doctor or nutritionist for nutritional guidance tailored to your personal and individual health needs.

CHAPTER 12
GROWING YOUR WELLNESS GARDEN

Transform your backyard into a healthy sanctuary by growing a healthy garden. Wellness Kitchen includes the concept "We taste good health" through the conscious cultivation of herbs, vegetables, and fruits that contribute not only to delicious dishes but also to your general well-being.

1. Conscious Planting

Start by choosing plants that are good for your health. Herbs like rosemary, basil, and mint can elevate your culinary creations by aiding digestion and reducing stress.

2. Nutrient-rich greens

Add nutrient-dense greens like kale, spinach, and Swiss chard to your garden. These vitamins and minerals add nutritional value to food and support a well-rounded diet.

3. Colorful selection

Combine different colorful vegetables and fruits such as tomatoes, peppers, and berries. Vibrant colors indicate an abundance of antioxidants, which are important for cellular health and immune system function.

4. Medicinal plants

Discover the world of herbs such as chamomile, lavender, and echinacea. Not only do they enhance the sensory experience, but they also offer natural treatments for common ailments and promote a holistic approach to wellness.

5. Aromatherapy Garden

Use fragrant herbs like lavender and thyme to create an aromatherapy garden. Calming scents can reduce stress and anxiety and turn your garden into a therapeutic space.

6. Seasonality

Plan for seasonal variation to ensure a consistent harvest. Embrace the changing seasons with crops like pumpkins in the fall and strawberries in the spring, providing versatile nutrients year-round.

7. Mindfulness exercises

Practice mindfulness when tending to your garden. Use all your senses - feel the soil, smell the grass, listen to the rustle of the leaves. This relationship with nature promotes mental well-being and a sense of peace.

8. Garden to table philosophy

Embrace the "garden to table" philosophy, gathering fresh produce for meals. This not only ensures optimal freshness and taste but also strengthens the bond between your health garden and your plate.

9. Community involvement

Consider sharing the joy of gardening with your community. Collaborate on wellness gardening projects, swap seeds or produce, and promote collective wellness.

10. Sustainable practices

Use sustainable gardening practices like composting and water conservation to create an ecologically healthy garden. Caring for the planet is consistent with the broader goal of promoting the health of both individuals and the planet.

By cultivating your wellness garden, you are not only cultivating healthy ingredients but also a lifestyle focused on health and awareness. The wellness kitchen encourages you to enjoy the goodness that comes from intentionally and carefully increasing your well-being.

THE JOY OF HOMEGROWN HERBS AND VEGETABLES

In the healthy kitchen, enjoying good health begins with the joy of home herbs and vegetables. Cultivating your garden not only adds fresh flavors to your food but also nourishes your well-being. Tending to herbs and vegetables and watching them bloom under your care creates a connection with nature and is a source of pure enjoyment.

 Homemade herbs like basil, rosemary, and thyme add to the culinary experience and give dishes a richness of aroma that their store-bought counterparts can't match. From juicy tomatoes to crunchy cucumbers, the vibrant colors and intense flavors of freshly harvested vegetables offer a wealth of nutrients that support your overall health.

Beyond the nutritional value, growing your herbs and vegetables is a therapeutic journey. Digging soil, planting seeds, and tending to plants are meditative activities that promote mental well-being. The simple act of picking herbs or picking vegetables from the garden brings a deep sense of fulfillment and connection to the earth.

 The Wellness Kitchen embraces the cycle of planting, growing, and harvesting as a holistic approach to good health. By growing your herbs and vegetables, you not only enjoy the goodness of organic produce, but you also create a sustainable and conscious relationship with your food. So let the joy of homegrown herbs and vegetables be your guide to a healthier and more fulfilling life at the Wellness Kitchen.

TIPS FOR CULTIVATING A WELLNESS GARDEN

In "The Wellness Kitchen: Savoring Good Health," creating a wellness garden is a delightful journey to nourish both body and soul. Here are some tips for maintaining a healthy garden:

1. Careful selection of plants
Choose plants known for their health benefits. Add herbs like basil, rosemary, and mint, which not only add flavor to food but also offer medicinal properties.

2. Color choice
Include a rainbow of fruits and vegetables in your garden. Different colors often indicate different nutrients, resulting in a visually appealing and nutritious harvest.

3. Create a peaceful space
Create a quiet corner in your garden for meditation or yoga. Surround it with fragrant flowers and soothing greenery to enhance the soothing atmosphere.

4. Pluck Edible Flowers
Integrate edible flowers such as nasturtiums, marigolds, or pansies. Not only do they add

aesthetic appeal, but they also add unique flavors and nutrients to your culinary endeavors.

5. Natural Aromatherapy

Plant aromatic herbs such as lavender and chamomile. Their scents can have a calming effect, turning your garden into a natural sanctuary for relaxation.

6. Natural Practices

Use organic gardening methods to avoid harmful chemicals. This ensures that your products are pesticide-free, promoting a healthier lifestyle.

7. Including fruit trees

Plant fruit trees such as apples, pears, or citrus. Freshly picked fruit is not only delicious but also provides vitamins and antioxidants necessary for well-being.

8. Conscious Immersion

Practice conscious watering to conserve resources. Consider drip irrigation systems or rainwater harvesting methods to keep your garden sustainable.

9. The garden-to-table experience

Promote a direct connection between your garden and kitchen. Harvesting and cooking with freshly picked ingredients increases the nutritional value of your food.

10. **Create social spaces**
Set up living areas to enjoy the garden with friends and family. Growing a healthy garden isn't just about plants; it means promoting relationships and common well-being.

Remember that a healthy garden is not only about the plants you grow but also about its purpose and care. If you use these tips, you will enjoy not only good health but also a holistic and enriching gardening experience.

CHAPTER 13
CONCLUSION: YOUR JOURNEY TO OPTIMAL WELL-BEING

In concluding your journey to optimal well-being with "The Wellness Kitchen: Savoring Good Health," it's essential to reflect on the transformative power of nourishing your body and mind through wholesome choices. As you've explored the culinary landscape of healthful eating, you've cultivated a deeper connection with the foods that fuel vitality.

Embrace the knowledge gained about balanced nutrition, mindful eating, and the harmonious interplay between different ingredients. Your journey has been more than a culinary adventure; it's been a conscious decision to prioritize your well-being. From vibrant fruits and vegetables to lean proteins and whole grains, each ingredient contributes to the symphony of wellness that resonates within you.

As you enjoy the flavors of good health, remember that wellness extends beyond the plate. A conscious approach to food in The Wellness Kitchen promotes a positive relationship with your body, emphasizing self-care and balance. Your new awareness will allow you to make informed choices that promote long-term health and happiness.

In this summary, celebrate those achievements, no matter how small, that has brought you closer to optimal well-being. Whether it's trying a new recipe, adopting healthier habits, or simply enjoying the joy of nourishing your body, every step is a win. As you continue this journey, let the lessons from "The Wellness Kitchen" be a guiding light toward sustained wellness, reminding you that good health is a lifelong commitment worth savoring.

RECAP OF YOUR WELLNESS KITCHEN ADVENTURE

The Wellness Kitchen was an amazing adventure that opened my eyes to the power of good nutrition and delicious food. From learning about the benefits of whole foods to trying new recipes, it has been a journey that has changed my life for the better.
Allow me to share a recap of my favorite moments from the Wellness Kitchen:
- Discover the power of superfoods and incorporate them into your daily diet.
- Learn about mindful eating and enjoying every bite.
- Researching new spices and herbs to improve flavors without adding unhealthy ingredients.
- Cooking with friends and family and sharing the joy of good food

Highlights of the Wellness Kitchen include:
- Finds ways to make cooking fun and efficient.
- Learn about different food cultures and traditions around the world.
- Understand the role of food in well-being and self-care.
- Share recipes and tips with others to spread the joy of healthy eating.

All in all, the Wellness Kitchen has been a journey of discovery and self-improvement. Focus on progress, not perfection. It's okay if you slip up or don't stick to your plan 100%. The key is progression and consistency over time. Focus on nutrition, not just calories. It's not just about eating less, it's about eating more nutritious foods that nourish your body.

Get creative in the kitchen. Have fun with food and try new recipes and ingredients. You might be surprised by what you find! Listen to your body. Pay attention to how you feel after eating certain foods, and here are a few more tips to help you get the most out of your Wellness Kitchen adventure. Make meal planning a priority. Set aside time each week to plan your meals and groceries. It makes healthy eating easier and more enjoyable.

Don't forget to drink water! Hydration is an important part of overall wellness. Incorporate movement into your day. Even a short walk can affect how you feel. Get enough sleep. Adequate rest is important for health and well-being. Reduces stress. Stress can hurt your health, so look for opportunities. More tips to help you create a wellness kitchen that works for you:

Don't forget gut health. The health of your gut is closely related to your overall health, so make sure you eat foods that support gut health. Consider intermittent fasting. Intermittent fasting has been shown to have health benefits such as weight loss and improved metabolism.

In conclusion, Wellness Kitchen is not only about what you eat but also about how you eat. Using the tips above, you can create a wellness kitchen that supports your health and well-being. Remember to focus on enjoying cooking and eating, and remember to listen to your body. Try it and enjoy! And remember that any small change can have a big impact on your overall well-being.

CHAPTER 14
APPENDIX: NUTRITIONAL INFORMATION AND REFERENCES

In Wellness Kitchen: Savoring Good Health, nutritional transparency is a priority to help you on your way to wellness. This supplement provides detailed nutritional information for the recipes in this cookbook and includes a comprehensive breakdown of calories, macronutrients, vitamins, and minerals.

NUTRITIONAL INFORMATION
(Per serving)

1. ***Breakfast Smoothie***
 -Calories: 180
- Protein: 15 g
- Carbohydrates: 25 g
- Fat: 5 g
- fiber: 8 g

2. ***Quinoa Power Bowl***
 Calories: 350
- Protein: 20 g
- Carbohydrates: 40 g
- Fat: 12 g
- fiber: 10 g

3. Chocolate All-Seed Pudding

 Calories: 200
- Protein: 12 g
- Carbohydrates: 30 g
- Fat: 8 g
- fiber: 12 g

4. Grilled Chicken Salad with Quinoa

- Calories: 320
- Protein: 28g
- Calcium: 15% of daily recommended intake
- Iron: Important for oxygen transport in the body.

REFERENCES

We have relied on reliable sources and scientific studies to ensure that the nutritional information provided is reliable. The nutritional content of this cookbook is based on the following references:

1. National Institute of Health (NIH) - Dietary Guidelines for Americans
2. Academy of Nutrition and Dietetic Sciences
3. World Health Organization (WHO) - Nutrition
4. Journal of the American Medical Association (JAMA).

These references are designed to guide you in making informed choices about your diet by promoting foods that not only taste good but also promote your health.

Note: Nutritional values are approximate and may vary depending on the ingredients used and portions. Ask your healthcare professional or registered dietitian for personalized nutritional advice tailored to your individual needs."

Feel free to modify the nutritional information based on specific recipes and information in The Wellness Kitchen: Tasting Good Health.